ASTHMA TREATMENT GUIDE FOR BEGINNERS

The Complete Guide On How To Cure, Get Rid And Manage Asthma Symptoms Through Diet Treatment

Vanessa Meza

Table of Contents

INTRODUCTION TO ASTHMA TREATMENTS

A. Definition And Overview Of Asthma

 B. Importance Of Effective Asthma Treatment

C. Purpose And Scope Of The Book

A. Definition and Overview of Asthma:

Start by defining asthma: Asthma is a chronic respiratory condition characterized by inflammation and narrowing of the airways, leading to symptoms such as wheezing, coughing, chest tightness, and shortness of breath.

Provide an overview of how asthma affects individuals: Asthma can vary in severity from mild to severe and can significantly impact a person's quality of life, daily activities, and even lead to life-threatening asthma attacks.

Explain the underlying causes of asthma: Asthma is often triggered by allergens, irritants, respiratory infections, exercise, or certain medications. It involves a complex interplay of genetic, environmental, and immune factors.

B. Importance of Effective Asthma Treatment:

Emphasize the importance of managing asthma effectively: Effective treatment and management of asthma are crucial for controlling symptoms, preventing exacerbations, and minimizing long-term complications.

Highlight the impact of uncontrolled asthma: Untreated or poorly managed asthma can lead to frequent hospitalizations, decreased lung function, missed school or work days, and diminished overall well-being.

Discuss the benefits of proper asthma management: Proper treatment can help individuals with asthma lead active, fulfilling lives, reduce the need for emergency medical care, and lower the risk of asthma-related mortality.

C. Purpose and Scope of the Book:

Explain the purpose of the book: The book aims to provide comprehensive information and guidance on asthma treatments to help patients, caregivers, and healthcare professionals better understand and manage the condition.

Outline the scope of the book: The book will cover various aspects of asthma treatment, including medications, inhaler techniques, lifestyle modifications, environmental control measures, and strategies for asthma management in different age groups and special populations.

Preview the content and organization: The book will be structured to provide clear and practical information, with chapters devoted to different treatment modalities, evidence-based guidelines, tips for self-management, and resources for further support.

CHAPTER ONE

UNDERSTANDING ASTHMA

A. Etiology And Pathophysiology Of Asthma

B. Types And Classification Of Asthma

C. Risk Factors And Triggers

A. Etiology and Pathophysiology of Asthma:

Define etiology and pathophysiology: Etiology refers to the cause or origin of a disease, while pathophysiology describes the abnormal physiological processes underlying the disease.

Explain the etiology of asthma: Asthma is a complex condition with multiple contributing factors, including genetic predisposition and environmental influences. It involves chronic inflammation of the airways, which leads to increased sensitivity and hyperresponsiveness to various triggers.

Describe the pathophysiology of asthma: In asthma, inflammation of the airways causes swelling, mucus production, and constriction of the smooth muscles surrounding the airways. This results in airflow obstruction and the characteristic symptoms of asthma, such as wheezing, coughing, and shortness of breath.

B. Types and Classification of Asthma:

Introduce the concept of asthma types and classification: Asthma is a heterogeneous disease with different phenotypes and clinical manifestations.

Discuss the classification of asthma based on severity: Asthma severity can be classified as intermittent, mild persistent, moderate persistent, or severe persistent, depending on the frequency and severity of symptoms and lung function measurements.

Explain the classification of asthma based on triggers: Asthma can also be classified based on triggers, such as allergic asthma (triggered by allergens like pollen, dust mites, or pet dander) or non-allergic asthma (triggered by irritants like smoke, pollution, or cold air).

C. Risk Factors and Triggers:

Define risk factors and triggers: Risk factors are factors that increase the likelihood of developing a disease, factors are factors that increase the likelihood of developing a disease, while triggers are factors that provoke asthma symptoms or exacerbations.

Discuss common risk factors for asthma: Risk factors for asthma include a family history of asthma or allergies, exposure to tobacco smoke during pregnancy or early childhood, respiratory infections, and certain environmental factors.

Identify common triggers for asthma: Asthma triggers can vary from person to person but may include allergens, respiratory infections, air pollution, smoke, exercise, cold air, and certain medications or chemicals.

DIAGNOSIS OF ASTHMA

A. Clinical Evaluation And History Taking

B. Physical Examination

C. Diagnostic Tests: Spirometry, Peak Flow Measurement, Allergy Testing, Imaging, Etc.

A. Clinical Evaluation and History Taking:

Begin with a comprehensive clinical evaluation: A healthcare provider will conduct a thorough assessment of the patient's medical history, including symptoms, frequency, and triggers of asthma-related episodes.

Emphasize the importance of history taking: Gathering information about the onset, duration, and progression of symptoms, as well as any family history of asthma or allergies, helps in establishing a diagnosis.

Discuss common asthma symptoms: Symptoms such as wheezing, coughing (especially at night or in response to triggers), shortness of breath, and chest tightness are indicative of asthma and should be explored during history taking.

B. Physical Examination: Highlight the role of physical examination: A healthcare provider will perform a physical examination to assess respiratory function and identify any signs of asthma or related complications.

Describe key findings during physical examination: Physical signs of asthma may include wheezing (audible upon auscultation of the chest), prolonged expiratory phase, increased respiratory rate, and use of accessory muscles for breathing.

Note that physical examination findings may vary depending on the severity and chronicity of asthma symptoms.

C. Diagnostic Tests:

Explain the importance of diagnostic tests: Diagnostic tests help confirm the diagnosis of asthma, assess lung function, identify triggers, and guide treatment decisions.

Discuss common diagnostic tests for asthma:

a. Spirometry: Spirometry measures lung function by assessing airflow obstruction and lung volumes. It is a key test for diagnosing and monitoring asthma. b. Peak flow measurement: Peak flow meters are portable devices used to measure peak expiratory flow rate, which can help assess the severity of airflow limitation and monitor asthma control.

c. Allergy testing: Allergy testing, such as skin prick tests or blood tests for specific IgE antibodies, can identify allergens that trigger asthma symptoms in allergic asthma.

d. Imaging: Imaging studies like chest X-rays or CT scans may be performed to evaluate lung function, assess airway inflammation, or rule out other respiratory conditions mimicking asthma.

Note that the combination of clinical evaluation, history taking, physical examination, and diagnostic tests is essential for an accurate diagnosis of asthma and for developing an individualized treatment plan.

CHAPTER TWO

CONVENTIONAL TREATMENT APPROACHES

A. Bronchodilators: Beta-Agonists and Anticholinergics:

Define bronchodilators: Bronchodilators are medications that work by relaxing the smooth muscles of the airways, leading to widening of the bronchioles and improved airflow.

Beta-agonists: Beta-agonists are a type of bronchodilator that stimulate beta-adrenergic receptors in the airway smooth muscles, causing relaxation. They are commonly used as quick-relief medications for acute asthma symptoms. Short-acting beta-agonists (SABAs) provide rapid relief during asthma attacks, while long-acting beta-agonists (LABAs) are used for long-term asthma control.

Anticholinergics: Anticholinergics are another type of bronchodilator that block the action of acetylcholine, a neurotransmitter that causes bronchoconstriction. They are often used as add-on therapy for moderate to severe asthma or as an alternative for individuals who cannot tolerate beta-agonists.

B. Anti-Inflammatory Medications: Corticosteroids, Leukotriene Modifiers, etc.:

Explain the role of anti-inflammatory medications: Anti-inflammatory medications help reduce airway inflammation, swelling, and mucus production, thereby preventing asthma symptoms and exacerbations.

Corticosteroids: Inhaled corticosteroids (ICS) are the most effective long-term control medications for asthma. They work by suppressing inflammation in the airways and reducing the frequency and severity of asthma symptoms. Oral corticosteroids may be used for short courses during severe asthma exacerbations.

Leukotriene modifiers: Leukotrienes are inflammatory mediators involved in asthma. Leukotriene modifiers, such as montelukast, zafirlukast, and zileuton, block the action of leukotrienes, thereby reducing inflammation, bronchoconstriction, and mucus secretion in the airways.

C. Combination Therapy:

Describe combination therapy: Combination therapy involves using two or more asthma medications with different mechanisms of action to achieve better asthma control and reduce the risk of exacerbations.

Combination inhalers: Combination inhalers contain both a corticosteroid and a long-acting beta-agonist (LABA) in a single device. They provide both anti-inflammatory and bronchodilator effects, making them convenient for patients with moderate to severe asthma.

Combination oral medications: In some cases, healthcare providers may prescribe a combination of different oral medications, such as an inhaled corticosteroid with a leukotriene modifier or a LABA.

D. Rescue Medications and Emergency Treatment:

Define rescue medications: Rescue medications, also known as quick-relief or short-acting medications, are used to provide rapid relief of asthma symptoms during acute exacerbations or asthma attacks.

Short-acting beta-agonists (SABAs): SABAs, such as albuterol and levalbuterol, are the most commonly used rescue medications. They quickly relieve bronchoconstriction and improve airflow within minutes.

Emergency treatment: In severe asthma exacerbations or life-threatening asthma attacks, emergency medical treatment may be necessary. This may include administration of high-dose inhaled or systemic corticosteroids, oxygen therapy, and in extreme cases, intubation and mechanical ventilation.

EMERGING THERAPEUTIC STRATEGIES

A. Biologic Therapies

B. Immunomodulators

C. Gene Therapy

D. Stem Cell Therapy

A. Biologic Therapies:

Define biologic therapies: Biologic therapies are a class of medications that target specific molecules or pathways involved in the inflammatory process underlying asthma.

Mechanism of action: Biologic therapies work by blocking cytokines or other molecules that play key roles in promoting inflammation and airway hyperresponsiveness in asthma.

Examples of biologic therapies: Biologic therapies approved for the treatment of severe asthma include monoclonal antibodies targeting interleukin (IL)-5 (e.g., mepolizumab, reslizumab, benralizumab), IL-4/IL-13 (e.g., dupilumab), and IgE (e.g., omalizumab). These medications are typically used as add-on therapy for patients with severe, uncontrolled asthma despite standard treatment.

B. Immunomodulators:

Explain immunomodulators: Immunomodulators are agents that modulate the immune system to restore balance and reduce inflammation in diseases such as asthma.

Mechanism of action: Immunomodulators may target various components of the immune system, including T cells, B cells, cytokines, or other immune cells involved in the pathogenesis of asthma.

Examples of immunomodulators: Emerging immunomodulatory therapies for asthma include small molecule inhibitors targeting specific signaling pathways involved in immune cell activation or cytokine production.

C. Gene Therapy:

Define gene therapy: Gene therapy is a therapeutic approach aimed at correcting genetic defects or modifying gene expression to treat or prevent diseases.

Potential application in asthma: Gene therapy for asthma aims to modulate the expression of genes involved in airway inflammation, hyperresponsiveness, or remodeling.

Current status: While gene therapy holds promise for the treatment of asthma, it is still in the experimental stage, and further research is needed to develop safe and effective gene delivery systems and to identify suitable gene targets for asthma treatment.

D. Stem Cell Therapy:

Explain stem cell therapy: Stem cell therapy involves the transplantation or manipulation of stem cells to repair damaged tissues or modulate immune responses in diseases like asthma.

Potential mechanisms of action: Stem cells have the potential to differentiate into various cell types, including airway epithelial cells, which could contribute to repair and regeneration of damaged airway tissues. Additionally, stem cells may exert immunomodulatory effects by suppressing inflammation and promoting tissue healing.

Clinical trials: Several clinical trials are exploring the safety and efficacy of stem cell therapy for asthma, including the use of mesenchymal stem cells (MSCs) derived from bone marrow or umbilical cord blood.

CHAPTER THREE

LIFESTYLE MANAGEMENT AND PREVENTIVE MEASURES

A. Identifying And Avoiding Triggers

B. Asthma Action Plans

C. Exercise And Physical Activity Recommendations

D. Dietary Considerations

A. Identifying and Avoiding Triggers:

Educate patients about common asthma triggers: Common triggers include allergens (e.g., pollen, dust mites, pet dander), irritants (e.g., smoke, pollution, strong odors), respiratory infections, cold air, exercise, and certain medications.

Encourage patients to identify their specific triggers: Keeping a diary to track symptoms and potential triggers can help patients identify patterns and avoid triggers that exacerbate their asthma.

Recommend strategies to minimize exposure: These may include using allergen-proof mattress and pillow covers, regularly cleaning and vacuuming the home, avoiding smoking or exposure to secondhand smoke, and using air purifiers or dehumidifiers to improve indoor air quality.

B. Asthma Action Plans:

Explain the importance of asthma action plans: Asthma action plans are personalized written instructions developed in collaboration with healthcare providers to help patients manage their asthma effectively.

Components of an asthma action plan: An asthma action plan typically includes instructions on daily medications, how to recognize and respond to worsening symptoms, when to seek medical help, and emergency contact information.

Encourage patients to carry and follow their action plans: Patients should keep their asthma action plans readily accessible and share them with family members, caregivers, teachers, and other relevant individuals.

C. Exercise and Physical Activity Recommendations:

Highlight the benefits of exercise for asthma management: Regular physical activity can improve lung function, cardiovascular health, and overall well-being in individuals with asthma.

Recommend appropriate exercise routines: Low to moderate intensity aerobic exercises such as walking, swimming, cycling, or yoga are generally well-tolerated by individuals with asthma.

Emphasize the importance of warm-up and cool-down: Patients should engage in proper warm-up and cool-down activities to minimize the risk of exercise-induced asthma symptoms.

Advise on using quick-relief medication before exercise: Patients with exercise-induced asthma may benefit from using a short-acting bronchodilator (e.g., albuterol) before engaging in physical activity to prevent symptoms.

D. Dietary Considerations:

Discuss the potential impact of diet on asthma: Certain dietary factors, such as omega-3 fatty acids, antioxidants, and vitamin D, may have anti-inflammatory properties and benefit individuals with asthma.

Encourage a balanced diet rich in fruits, vegetables, and whole grains: A diet high in fruits, vegetables, and whole grains provides essential nutrients and antioxidants that may help reduce inflammation and support overall lung health.

Consider potential food triggers: Some individuals with asthma may have food allergies or sensitivities that can trigger asthma symptoms. It may be helpful to identify and avoid these triggers through allergy testing or elimination diets.

CHAPTER FOUR

COMPLEMENTARY AND ALTERNATIVE THERAPIES

A. Herbal Remedies And Supplements

B. Acupuncture

C. Breathing Techniques: Yoga, Tai Chi, Etc.

D. Chiropractic Care

A. Herbal Remedies and Supplements:

Discuss the use of herbal remedies:

Some individuals with asthma may use herbal remedies or dietary supplements in an attempt to manage their symptoms or reduce inflammation.

Common herbal remedies: Examples include herbal teas (e.g., chamomile, ginger), herbal extracts (e.g., boswellia, butterbur), and traditional Chinese herbs (e.g., ma huang, licorice root).

Caution regarding herbal remedies: While some herbal remedies may have anecdotal evidence supporting their use for asthma, scientific research on their safety and effectiveness is often limited. Patients should exercise caution and consult with their healthcare provider before using herbal remedies, as they may interact with medications or exacerbate asthma symptoms in some cases.

B. Acupuncture:

Explain acupuncture: Acupuncture is a traditional Chinese medicine practice involving the insertion of thin needles into specific points on the body to stimulate energy flow (Qi) and restore balance.

Potential benefits for asthma: Some studies suggest that acupuncture may help reduce asthma symptoms, improve lung function, and enhance quality of life in individuals with asthma by modulating immune responses, reducing inflammation, and promoting relaxation.

Limited evidence and individual response: While acupuncture may offer benefits for some individuals with asthma, the evidence supporting its efficacy is mixed, and individual responses may vary. More research is needed to fully understand its role in asthma management.

C. Breathing Techniques: Yoga, Tai Chi, etc.:

Discuss breathing techniques: Breathing techniques such as yoga, tai chi, qigong, and mindfulness-based practices emphasize controlled breathing patterns, relaxation, and mind-body awareness.

Potential benefits for asthma: Breathing techniques may help individuals with asthma improve lung function, reduce stress, and manage anxiety associated with asthma symptoms. They can also enhance respiratory muscle strength and control.

Incorporating breathing exercises into asthma management: Patients can learn and practice breathing exercises as part of their asthma self-management plan. These techniques can complement conventional asthma treatments and provide additional tools for symptom relief and stress management.

D. Chiropractic Care:

Describe chiropractic care: Chiropractic care involves manual manipulation of the spine and musculoskeletal system to improve alignment, mobility, and nervous system function.

Limited evidence for asthma: While some chiropractors may claim that spinal manipulation can improve asthma symptoms by restoring nerve function and immune responses, scientific evidence supporting the effectiveness of chiropractic care for asthma is lacking.

Safety considerations: Individuals considering chiropractic care for asthma should consult with their healthcare provider and ensure that the chiropractor is qualified and experienced in treating asthma or respiratory conditions. They should also be aware of potential risks and contraindications associated with spinal manipulation.

SPECIAL CONSIDERATIONS

A. Asthma In Children: Diagnosis And Treatment

B. Asthma In Pregnancy

C. Occupational Asthma

D. Severe Asthma And Difficult-To-Treat Cases

A. Asthma in Children: Diagnosis and Treatment:

Diagnosis: Asthma in children can be challenging to diagnose due to overlapping symptoms with other respiratory conditions and limitations in performing lung function tests.

Diagnosis typically relies on clinical evaluation, medical history, and assessment of response to asthma medications.

Treatment: Asthma management in children involves a combination of preventive measures (e.g., identifying and avoiding triggers), daily controller medications (e.g., inhaled corticosteroids), and rescue medications (e.g., short-acting beta-agonists) as needed. Education and involvement of parents and caregivers are crucial for successful asthma management in children.

B. Asthma in Pregnancy:

Diagnosis and monitoring: Asthma management during pregnancy requires careful monitoring and adjustment of medications to ensure optimal control while minimizing risks to the mother and fetus. Regular prenatal visits with healthcare providers are essential for assessing asthma control and adjusting treatment as needed.

Medication considerations: In general, inhaled corticosteroids are considered safe and effective for asthma management during pregnancy and should be continued as prescribed to maintain asthma control. Other asthma medications, such as short-acting beta-agonists and oral corticosteroids, may be used as needed under the guidance of healthcare providers.

C. Occupational Asthma:

Definition: Occupational asthma refers to asthma that is caused or exacerbated by exposure to allergens or irritants in the workplace environment.

Diagnosis: Diagnosis of occupational asthma involves identifying a temporal relationship between work exposure and onset or worsening of asthma symptoms, as well as confirming the presence of airway hyperresponsiveness or inflammation through objective tests such as spirometry or bronchial challenge tests.

Management: Management of occupational asthma includes identifying and reducing exposure to workplace triggers, providing appropriate respiratory protection, and considering job modification or relocation if necessary. Early recognition and intervention are crucial to prevent progression and long-term disability.

D. Severe Asthma and Difficult-to-Treat Cases:

Definition: Severe asthma refers to asthma that remains uncontrolled despite high-dose treatment with inhaled corticosteroids and other controller medications. Difficult-to-treat asthma encompasses both severe asthma and cases where asthma control is not achieved despite adherence to treatment.

Evaluation and management: Evaluation of severe asthma requires comprehensive assessment to identify contributing factors such as comorbidities, medication adherence, environmental exposures, and psychosocial factors. Treatment of severe asthma may involve higher doses of controller medications, biologic therapies, and multidisciplinary care involving pulmonologists, allergists, and other specialists.

CHAPTER FIVE

PATIENT EDUCATION AND EMPOWERMENT

A. Importance Of Asthma Education

B. Self-Management Techniques

C. Resources And Support Groups

A. Importance of Asthma Education:

Understanding the condition: Asthma education helps patients and their families understand the nature of asthma, including its causes, symptoms, triggers, and underlying mechanisms.

Treatment options: Educating patients about available treatment options, including medications, inhaler techniques, and lifestyle modifications, empowers them to actively participate in their asthma management.

Asthma action plans: Asthma education includes developing personalized asthma action plans in collaboration with healthcare providers. These plans provide clear instructions on daily medications, recognizing and managing symptoms, and when to seek medical help or emergency care.

Prevention of exacerbations: Educating patients about identifying and avoiding asthma triggers, practicing proper medication adherence, and recognizing early warning signs of worsening symptoms can help prevent asthma exacerbations and improve overall asthma control.

B. Self-Management Techniques: Medication adherence: Teaching patients the importance of taking their prescribed medications regularly and correctly, including both controller and rescue medications, is crucial for maintaining asthma control.

Inhaler techniques: Proper inhaler technique ensures optimal delivery of medication to the lungs. Patients should receive hands-on training from healthcare providers on how to use their inhalers correctly and regularly review their technique to ensure efficacy.

Monitoring symptoms: Encouraging patients to monitor their asthma symptoms and peak flow measurements regularly helps track asthma control and detect changes or worsening symptoms promptly.

Lifestyle modifications: Providing guidance on lifestyle modifications, such as avoiding tobacco smoke, maintaining a healthy weight, managing stress, and incorporating regular exercise, supports overall asthma management and improves quality of life.

C. Resources and Support Groups: Healthcare provider support: Patients should feel comfortable discussing their asthma concerns, questions, and treatment goals with their healthcare providers. Regular follow-up visits allow for ongoing monitoring, adjustment of treatment plans, and addressing any barriers to asthma management.

Patient education materials: Providing patients with educational materials, such as pamphlets, brochures, or online resources, reinforces key asthma management concepts and empowers them to make informed decisions about their health.

Support groups: Connecting patients with asthma support groups or online communities allows them to share experiences, tips, and coping strategies with others facing similar challenges.

Peer support can provide valuable emotional support and motivation for managing asthma effectively.

CHAPTER SIX

FUTURE DIRECTIONS AND INNOVATIONS IN ASTHMA TREATMENT

A. Advances In Precision Medicine

B. Personalized Treatment Approaches

C. Potential Cure Research

A. Advances in Precision Medicine:

Definition: Precision medicine aims to tailor medical treatment and interventions to individual patients based on their unique genetic, environmental, and lifestyle factors.

Application in asthma: Advances in precision medicine hold promise for identifying specific asthma phenotypes and endotypes, enabling targeted therapies that address underlying molecular pathways and immune mechanisms driving asthma.

Biomarkers and targeted therapies: Biomarkers such as blood eosinophil counts, fractional exhaled nitric oxide (FeNO) levels, and specific IgE antibodies help identify patients who may benefit from biologic therapies targeting cytokines or immunoglobulins involved in asthma inflammation.

B. Personalized Treatment Approaches:

Individualized treatment plans: Personalized treatment approaches consider factors such as asthma severity, triggers, comorbidities, medication responses, and patient preferences to develop tailored asthma management plans.

Pharmacogenomics:

Pharmacogenomic testing can help identify genetic variations that influence drug metabolism and response, guiding the selection of the most effective and safest asthma medications for individual patients.

Digital health technologies: Wearable devices, smartphone applications, and electronic health records facilitate remote monitoring of asthma symptoms, medication adherence, and lung function, enabling real-time adjustments to treatment plans based on individual patient data.

C. Potential Cure Research:

Gene therapy: Gene editing technologies such as CRISPR/Cas9 hold promise for correcting genetic mutations associated with asthma susceptibility or severity, potentially offering a curative approach for select individuals with monogenic forms of asthma.

Immunomodulation: Research into novel immunomodulatory agents and immune tolerance induction strategies aims to reset dysregulated immune responses in asthma, potentially leading to long-term remission or cure.

Stem cell therapy: Stem cell-based approaches for airway regeneration and immune modulation offer potential avenues for restoring normal lung structure and function in individuals with severe asthma or airway remodeling.

CONCLUSION

A. Recap of Key Points:

Throughout this discussion, we've explored various aspects of asthma diagnosis, treatment, and management. We've covered the definition and overview of asthma, the importance of effective treatment, conventional and emerging therapeutic approaches, lifestyle management and preventive measures, special considerations, patient education and empowerment, and future directions in asthma treatment.

B. Encouragement for Patients and Caregivers:

For patients and caregivers facing the challenges of asthma, it's important to remember that asthma can be effectively managed with proper education, treatment, and support. By working closely with healthcare providers, following personalized treatment plans, and implementing lifestyle modifications, individuals with asthma can achieve better control over their symptoms and improve their quality of life. It's essential to stay proactive, advocate for your health needs, and seek help when needed.

C. Hope for the Future of Asthma Treatment:

The future of asthma treatment holds promise for continued advancements in precision medicine, personalized treatment approaches, and potential cures. With ongoing research and innovation, we are moving closer to identifying the underlying mechanisms of asthma, developing targeted therapies, and ultimately finding ways to prevent or cure this chronic respiratory condition. While challenges remain, there is reason to be hopeful for the future of asthma treatment and the prospect of improved outcomes for patients worldwide.

THE END